Agonizing stretch marks

How To Get Rid Of Stretch Marks:Natural Cures and Remedies
For Stretch Marks

Lisa Drake

Published By

Lisa Drake

Copyright @ 2014

What are these things called Stretch

Marks

No one likes getting . They are unsightly and they never really go away. Ironically though, everyone can get them. People of all ages, races and genders can get stretch marks although they are more common among women and particularly common among pregnant women, with 9 out of 10 women getting them. So what are they, what causes them and how can we avoid them? Any discussion about stretch marks will have to begin with an explanation of exactly what they are.

There are varying explanations of how and why stretch marks are formed.

1. Stretch marks or Straie, are caused when the middle layer of the skin or the dermis is torn allowing the inner layers to show through. This happens when the skin's elasticity breaks down. The stretching causes the connective tissue to break down leading to inflammation. There is microscopic bleeding that shows up as red or purple and later scarring. It is the scars that cause the marks. When the under layer stretches the epidermis also stretches and allows the layer underneath to be visible. They take the form of long, narrow streaks or lines that develop on the surface of the skin. Stretch marks usually occur when the skin goes through rapid stretching such as in the case of pregnancy or when there is rapid growth or what is called a growth spurt such as what is experienced by some children and teenagers. The rapid increase in muscle mass that is caused by body building also leads to stretch marks.

2. Recent studies have led some researchers to believe that stretching of the skin is not the total cause of stretch marks. They believe that it is also the hormones that are released when a person gains or loses a great deal of weight or is pregnant or going through the teen years, that lead to the formation of stretch marks. If the stretching is accompanied by an increase in the production of the hormone cortisone by the adrenal gland the stretch marks appear more pronounced. That is because cortisone causes the fiber in the skin to be less elastic.

3. Research has found that the use of steroids through ingestion as either with pills or topical application as with lotions and creams can also lead to stretch marks. Some studies suggest that there is a link between stress and development of stretch marks. The two are linked by the steroid cortisol which the body releases when it experiences stress. The presence of stress makes the body think it is at risk and it therefore goes into survival mode which includes storing fat so that there is rapid weight gain which in turn leads to stretch marks.

4. If you are suffering from diseases such as Cushing's Syndrome, Adrenal Gland Disease or any inherited genetic disorders you will be predisposed to develop stretch marks.

Stretch marks can occur anywhere on the body but they are most commonly found in areas that have large deposits of fat such as the stomach, breasts, thighs or buttocks. The look of stretch marks depends on several factors including how long you have had them, where they are located and what caused them. Some marks look like long indentations in the skin while others are pink, red or purple streaks and yet others have faded to white or gray. Over time they fade to a lighter color, they do not endanger a person's health in any way and they do fade over time. Their appearance will also depend on the type of skin that you have. People with more melanin are less likely to get stretch marks than people who have little melanin in their skin. Melanin is the pigment found in the epidermis and is produced by cells known as melanocytes. It determines the specific color of the skin.

There are certain things that predispose a person to developing stretch marks

1. Gender – women are more likely to develop stretch marks than men

2. Genetics- If there is a history of stretch marks in your family e.g. if you mother and aunt had them then you are more likely to get them.

3. Pregnancy – stretch marks are very common in pregnant women and even more so in young mothers to be. Giving birth to a big baby or having multiple births increases the risk further

4. Puberty

5. Obesity- overweight people are more likely to have stretch marks that those who maintain a healthy weight

6. Rapid weight gain or weight loss.

7. The presence of certain ailments.

There are also some indicators that stretch marks are going to appear. Most people say that the skin starts to itch before the marks appear. The skin will also often appear thinner and depending on your skin color it may turn pink. The lines when they come in will be slightly raised and the skin will be wrinkled. Be careful not to itch the area as scratching stretches the skin and will make things worse. Massage the area instead using cream, oil or lotion as massage helps the circulation as well as stopping the itching. It also encourages the growth of new cells which results in faster healing.

How to Avoid Getting Stretcsh Mark

Many people try to prevent the development of stretch marks by using topical creams and lotions before they appear but there is no real evidence to suggest that these creams work. However, there are some things that can to be done to lower the risk of getting these ugly marks.

1. **Perhaps the most important thing to do if you want to avoid stretch marks is to maintain a healthy weight.** Avoid fad diets that cause your weight to fluctuate greatly over a short period of time as sudden weight gain and/or loss often lead to stretch marks. If you need to lose weight do so slowly through eating a healthy diet and exercising. Try not to lose more than 1lb per week.

2. **Care for your skin.** Massage your skin with moisturizers every day, twice a day. Stretch marks are much more common among people with dry skin. Use steady pressure and work in a circular motion for 2 to 3 minutes. Massage also helps the circulation and stimulates the growth of new tissue. In order to have healthy skin it is also important to eat a healthy diet. Eat food that is good for your skin. Ensure that your diet is rich in Vitamins, especially A, E, and C, and minerals because this helps in keeping the skin supple.

3. **Keep your skin hydrated.** You should drink a lot of water. The more active you are the more water you need. Some medical professionals recommend drinking at least 64 ozs of

water per day. Remember not to drink it all at once though because the body will expel whatever it doesn't need at that time. If you drink enough water it will help your skin to maintain its elasticity and if it is elastic it will be less likely to tear when it stretches. Drinking water also helps you to cut down on how much you eat so it helps in avoiding weight gain.

4. **Manage your pregnancy.** During your pregnancy do not be tempted to overeat just because you are pregnant. The baby does not need that second cupcake to survive. Eat the right foods from as many of the food groups as possible. Try to keep your weight gain slow and gradual. If you were a fairly average weight before you got pregnant you should try to keep your weight gain between 25-30 lbs. during the course of your pregnancy. If you were underweight then it's okay to gain a little more and if you were overweight you should try not to gain any more than 20 extra lbs.

5. **Use Moisturizing creams.** Creams such as Vitamin E oil help to heal skin so they can greatly reduce the appearance of stretch mark if they are caught really early or as they are just beginning to form. There are many of these creams on the market so be sure to read the labels carefully and do your research before purchasing and applying them. Look for creams that contain peptides. Scar treatment cream has been reported to be effective in reducing the appearance of stretch marks. Cocoa butter creams are also a favorite. If you moisturize your skin regularly it will maintain its elasticity longer and be able to stretch without stretch marks forming. There are many natural moisturizers that you can use such as olive oil, almond oil, coconut oil, or tea tree oil.

6. **Exercise.** Exercise is good for the body and what is good for the body is good for the skin. Cardio healthy routines help circulation which is also good for keeping the skin supple. If weight lifting is part of your regular routine be careful not to build muscle too quickly as this is a recipe for stretch marks.

7. **Stretch.** If you add a stretching routine to your regular exercise regimen this will add elasticity to your skin.

8. **Do not scratch.** If your skin feels itchy especially in areas where stretch marks would commonly appear, massage the area with oils and creams but do not scratch the skin as

this can lead to the appearance of stretch marks. Examples of problem areas would be the thighs and hip, the breasts and the stomach. If you need help finding the right creams to use consult your physician.

Is it Possible to Get Rid of Stretch

Marks?

Although there have been numerous remedies for stretch marks advertised and talked about, none of them seem to work that well. There are some treatments that do have a degree of success and how well they work depends on the age of the person who has the stretch marks as well as that person's skin tone and even diet. It is also important to start treating your stretch marks as soon as they appear as when they begin to flatten they are harder to treat.

Here are some of the more common remedies

1. **To improve your blood circulation**, take hot baths or showers and massage the affected area. This will accelerate the healing process.

2. **Prescription medication**- Tretinoin creams such as Retin A are particularly helpful in improving the look of recent stretch marks although they do not have much effect on

older marks and they only show results if the dosage is high and the creams are applied over a significant period of time. These creams are retinoids so they make the skin thicker. These creams are not recommended for pregnant women or for nursing mothers and should be used under the direction of a medical doctor. What the cream does is rebuild collagen in the skin so that the stretch mark becomes less noticeable. There are a few side effects in that the cream can irritate your skin. Get the prescription from your dermatologist.

3. **Laser therapy**- this type of therapy involves the use of intense wavelengths of light to increase collagen or Elastin growth or the production of melanin in the skin. Different lasers are used depending on the type of stretch mark.

The most common types of laser treatment are:

Pulsed dye laser – this type of laser treatment has the best results on recent stretch marks.

Fractional laser – this type is more successful with older stretch marks that have turned white or gray. This type of laser makes tiny cuts where the stretch marks are and leaves normal skin in between them. The body heals the treated area with healthy new skin. Overtime the marks shrink and the skin tightens and appears smoother. This treatment stimulates the production of collagen and healthy tissue. It takes about three sessions and is quite expensive. It should be noted that fractional laser treatments are not recommended for people with very dark skin so find out from your medical practitioner beforehand whether or not you are a suitable candidate.

Vascular laser – Vascular laser treatment reduces the inflammation of the skin that accompanies stretch marks and in so doing prevents the skin from being damaged any further and stops the marks from getting any worse.

Laser treatment is not really painful but there is discomfort. There are several drawbacks to using this type of treatment:

i.   You will need more than one treatment and the whole process can take quite some time.

ii.   Laser therapy can get quite expensive

iii.   Laser therapy doesn't repair damaged tissue

iv.   The treatment results in swelling and redness, sometimes there are blisters and bruising as well and there might be changes in pigmentation

v.   Laser treatment is considered cosmetic and so is hardly ever covered by health insurance.

Laser therapy doesn't interfere with a person's normal routine in anyway even though it may take a few days for the swelling to go down. Fair skinned people tend to see better results from this type of treatment than others and you should not use it if your family has a history of Vitiligo or hyperventilation. You should always get a skin evaluation before trying this type of therapy under the supervision of a dermatologist or cosmetic doctor. There is a risk that scarring might occur.

4. **Another form of treatment for stretch marks is Intense Pulsed Light or IPL**. This treatment reduces the color difference between the stretch marks and the rest of your skin, thereby making the marks less noticeable. This treatment doesn't treat the change in skin texture that occurs when you get stretch marks.

5. **Over the counter creams and lotions**- these are not very effective although moisturizing does help because it reduces the itching that often accompanies stretch marks and can also improve their appearance. To remove stretch marks you will need to use natural oils as the creams with artificial ingredients are not effective. Find a product that penetrates to the second layer of the skin so that they can affect the stretch marks where they are formed. The creams should contain ingredients such as Aloe Vera, Vitamin E or Jojoba oil. Again you should consult a dermatologist or cosmetic surgeon before taking any over the counter drugs. Shea butter moisturizes the skin and reduces the appearance of stretch marks and helps to keep them away. Use the butter twice a day but be patient because it takes several weeks before any effect can be seen. Another option involves rubbing Vitamin e gel into the skin every day for at least two weeks.

6. **Micro-dermabrasion**- This involves the use of a hand-held machine that blows crystals unto the skin. The Crystals wear away the top layer of dead skin, polishing the surface.

The crystals and the skin cells they remove are then sucked into a vacuum tube. What this achieves is the removal of the top layer of skin and in turn this activates new growth. The new skin will be more elastic than the skin it replaced. The skin tone and texture will be improved. This type of treatment is recommended for older stretch marks. It needs about 3 sessions for the marks to be less noticeable. The problem is it doesn't go deep enough to really affect the stretch marks.

7. **Chemical Peels** – Peels remove the skin's top layer and this helps the marks to look less discolored. If you decide to have a peel you should get it done by a dermatologist if you want the best results. Chemical peels are not really recommended as a way of dealing with stretch marks.

8. **Surgery** – When having a tummy tuck or breast implants or reduction you can use that opportunity to remove the marks when you are removing other areas of skin. With a tummy tuck you probably get the best results because the skin is removed all together. People who gain and then lose a great deal of weight very quickly usually develop very bad stretch marks and so sometimes consider a tummy tuck as an option. This is a very expensive option and it leaves a scar. Surgery is not recommended as a way of getting rid of stretch marks.

9. **Diet-** this has to be done before the stretch marks develop. Eating healthy helps you to avoid rapid weight gain which is one of the occurrences that lead to stretch marks.

10. **Exfoliation** – when taking a bath use a loofah to gently scrub the skin in the area of the stretch marks to remove the dead skin and so minimize the appearance of the stretch marks.

11. **Endermologie-** This involves cell mechanical stimulation and would be performed by a dermatologist or other skin professional using machines called rollers and a vacuuming machine which softens the skin. The mechanical stimulation is thought to cause the cells to produce collagen and elastin. This technique was first developed by the French plastic surgeon Louis Pal Guitay. Reported to feel like deep tissue massage, it is said to be painless and is also used to rid patients of cellulite. If you are to see the effects of this

technique several sessions will be required each one lasting about 45 minutes. When the cost of all the session is calculated this treatment can be quite expensive.

The most common side effect of this treatment is bruising of the skin.

12. **Alpha Hydroxy Acids**. Alpha Hydroxy acids are believed to penetrate and dissolve dead skin. This allows for the new skin underneath to be exposed. These acids occur naturally in fruits and are found in high concentration in fruits such as pineapple, papayas and all kinds of citrus fruits. They can also be produced synthetically and are used in products that exfoliate the skin or in chemical peels. If you do not want to use the commercial or synthetic products you can simply rub the skin of the fruit on your face. You have to be careful when using this method because of the concentration of the acid is very high it can damage the skin causing redness and in extreme cases oozing. When you use a product that contains Alpha Hydroxy Acid for the first time it is a good idea to do a skin test on a small patch of skin first and if you go out in the sun after using a peel or micro-abrasion on your skin please be sure to use sunscreen with a very high SPF to protect the new skin.

If you want to avoid paying the high cost of commercial products that contain these acids, you can make your own alpha hydroxyl acid by combining raw brown sugar and the juice of grapes that are not yet ripe then mixing the two ingredients in an oil that comes from a plant such as coconut or jojoba oil. This will produce glycolic acid which is a form of Alpha Hydroxy Acid. Mix the ingredients into a paste and apply it to the affected area, leaving it on for 15-20 minutes before rinsing it off. Routine applications of the paste over time will give the desired results. Glycolic Acid and Vitamin C when combined and applied to the skin over a period of time appear to have the effect of fading stretch marks.

Another way of making Alpha Hydroxy Acid is mixing apple cider vinegar and water. Apples produce malic acid which is very effective in dissolving dead skin cells. Apply the mixture to the stretch marks with a cotton swab regularly; leave on for about 10 minutes, then rinse.

It should be noted that none of these remedies are 100% successful because they do not rid the recipient of stretch marks completely. It is also important to note that laser treatment, microdermabrasion and tummy tucks are all very expensive. It also true thought that most people are happy to fade the marks to white or grey and then forget about them.

For fading Stretch marks you can also try Shea butter. It moisturizes and reduces the appearance of stretch marks and helps keep them away. Use the Shea butter twice a day but be patient it takes weeks before its effects can be seen. You can also use baby oil and olive oil to fade stretch marks.

Natural Remedies for Removing

Stretch Marks

1. Vera: - Even if you put aside the use of Aloe Vera for removing stretch marks Aloe Vera is still very good for you because it is loaded with vitamins and minerals. It also has plant collagen and this goes deep into the skin and provides nourishment. Aloe Vera is an antibiotic and an anesthetic. It hydrates and promotes the growth of cells. It helps skin to

retain its moisture and promotes the production of elastin and collagen. Aloe Vera helps the skin to thicken and therefore reduce the appearance of stretch marks.

Apply the Aloe Vera cream to the skin every morning. It gets absorbed by the skin so it gets to the dermis. If it is applied before the stretch marks are formed e.g. in the early stages of pregnancy as the skin on the abdomen begins to stretch this is when the cream is most effective. If, however, the marks have already been formed it might take months for you to see real results.

Aloe Vera is a natural product so there are no unwanted chemicals in the cream. Aloe Vera is an antibiotic and anesthetic, and is known to promote cell growth. Aloe Vera also has vitamins and minerals and it helps the skin to retain moisture. It also it also helps the skin. There are, however, people who are allergic to the aloe plant so if you find that your skin begins to itch when you apply the cream then you might want to discontinue use. It should be noted though that some people have found that the side effects are only temporary.

2. Vitamin E -Massage Vitamin E oil into the affected area. This is thought to promote the growth of skin that is healthy. Pure Vitamin e oil that has no chemicals is a natural way to increase the elasticity of your skin. Vitamin e oil is rich in antioxidants and these regulate the cells in the skin as well as protecting it from the UV rays of the sun which make stretch marks look worse. It accelerates healing of the skin and regeneration. The essential fatty acids in the oil assist in absorption of the Vitamin e into the skin.

   If you aren't using the oil you can get your vitamin e from foods such as eggs, nuts and vegetable oils but applying the oil directly to the problem area is much more effective

3. You can also mix Vitamin A ointment with Vitamin E oil and apply to the skin, leaving on for about half an hour before rinsing and cleaning. This would have to be done consistently for several weeks before you notice any results.

4. Massage coconut oil mixed with lime juice and cocoa butter into the skin daily. Some people have reported a marked difference in the appearance of their skin in a short period of time. Coconut is thought to improve elastin fibers in the skin which helps to reduce the incidence and appearance of stretch marks. It is better to apply the mixture to wet skin

because absorption is better. Pat yourself dry afterward so the mixture doesn't get rubbed off.

5. Mix coffee, bicarbonate of soda, vitamin E oil and cocoa butter and use it as an exfoliate for the skin. Do this twice a day. Apart from removing dead skin cells it helps the Vitamin E and cocoa butter to be absorbed into the skin.

6. Make a paste out of water, baking soda, cocoa butter and Vitamin e oil. Apply to the skin regularly and leave on for 20-30 minutes.

7. Make a mixture of Olive Oil, aloe Vera Gel, the liquid of 6 Vitamin e capsules and 4 Vitamin A capsules and apply to the skin daily. Keep the excess lotion refrigerated.

8. Make a homemade moisturizer out of Vitamin E oil, cocoa butter and Vitamin C powder. Use it on the skin after using a natural exfoliation such as the one above.

9. Apply lemon juice to your skin and leave it to dry. When it has dried cover the area with Aloe Vera and leave it on overnight. Rinse the cream and juice off the next morning. Repeat this every night.

10. Make a scrub out of salt, honey and glycerin (about ½ tsp of salt to 1 sp of honey). Mix and massage the mixture into the area that has the stretch marks. Leave on for a few minutes then rinse with warm water and gently clean the area.

11. Mix ½ a carrot with the peel of a tangerine, 4 tablespoons of olive oil in a blender. Massage the mixture into wet skin after a bath or shower then rinse and pat dry. Repeat as often as possible.

12. Ascorbic Acid or Vitamin C increases the collagen production in the body and in so doing reduces the appearance of stretch marks. Crush a tablet or two and apply to the skin twice a day.

13. To improve blood circulation massage the affected area whenever taking a hot shower or bath. This will accelerate the healing process.

14. Rub Vitamin E gel into the skin for at least 2 weeks.

Some of these natural remedies must be applied regularly over a long period of time before the results can really be seen so if you are going the natural route be prepared to be patient. How long it actually takes and the degree of success that you have will depend on the type of skin that you have and the severity of the stretch marks.

Alternative cures for Stretch marks

There are also remedies for stretch marks in the field of alternative medicine. Here are some of the options available for persons who don't want to use synthetic materials.

Gotu Kola- Gotu Kola is a plant extract that was used in ancient Chinese herbal medicine. It has also been used in India and Indonesia. The plant has been found growing in India, Sri Lanka, Madagascar, South America and in the Tropics. This plant is thought to have skin repair properties and is often used in the production of skin care products. It has been shown to improve circulation and heal wounds and that is why it is used to prevent and treat stretch marks. Also known as Centella Asiatica, the plant is eaten in Sri Lanka with rice and curry. It is an antibacterial and anti-inflammatory but it is its ability to heal wounds that makes it the herb of choice for treating stretch marks.

Tips on How to Cover Up Stretch marks

1. Make Up: there is a type of foundation used by models that really qualifies as body make up and which is thicker than normal make up. Apply this to the skin will mask stretch marks.

2. Tattoos: Putting a tattoo over an area that you have stretch marks in can mask the marks. Of course a tattoo is as permanent as the stretch marks are so think carefully before making the commitment. A good compromise is to get temporary tattoos just for the times when you are worried about your stretch marks showing.

3. Air-brushing – this covers all stretch marks and lasts for about 12 hours before it begins to fade and it needs regular touch ups. Try to match your skin tone as closely as possible.

4. Combine bronzer and cocoa butter and apply to stretch marks. The cocoa butter helps the skin to heal and the bronzer covers the marks. Blend the mixture into the stretch marks and let it dry. Once dry apply some translucent powder to set so it won't rub off on your clothes.

5. Sunless tanning creams and lotions help in masking the appearance of stretch marks do not use tanning beds however because stretch marks do not tan and might become even more noticeable.

6. Stay away from clothes that expose your stretch marks if they embarrass you. If there are stretch marks on your stomach or thighs avoid short shorts, crop tops and bikinis. For women who are embarrassed by their stretch marks when at the pool or beach, you can always go for the currently fashionable one-piece swimsuit or a 'tankini' that covers the stomach. Move around a lot when you try it on to see if it shifts and exposes the marks you are trying to hide. You can also wear a beach wrap in one of the many fashionable styles that are now available to cover your problem area.

NB Natural tanning does not work to hide stretch marks.

Pregnancy and Stretch Marks

some people it is impossible to prevent stretch marks during pregnancy. Studies have shown that roughly 80% of women will develop stretch marks during this period especially in the final trimester when the growth of the fetus is rapid. No one can tell who will get them and who won't but one thing is certain, an expectant mother will gain weight and she will do so in a relatively short period of time. Over the years studies have indicated that younger women have a higher incidence of stretch marks than older mothers. Stretch marks that develop during pregnancy tend to be on the abdomen but they also show up on the breasts, thighs, lower back and buttocks. If you had them with a previous pregnancy chances are you will have them again although it might not be new ones but just the ones that were already there darkening again and possibly getting wider.

Apart from the rapid weight gain during pregnancy the body also produces hormones that act as softeners for the fibers in your skin and as a result of this the skin becomes more prone to developing stretch marks. The stretch marks that appear on a woman's abdomen when pregnant are usually dark colored. Although the stretch marks will fade once the baby is born they will not disappear completely.

There are several things that expectant mothers can do to cut the risk of developing stretch marks. Even if they don't work they will at least keep your skin moisturized and reduce itching. Pregnant women can use Vitamin e treatments once a day in the early stages of their pregnancy to keep their skin soft and supple and twice a day as the delivery approaches. For the best results mothers-to-be are encouraged to massage the Vitamin e oil into the stomach area. Almond oil can also be used during pregnancy to keep skin soft and ward off the appearance of stretch marks. It strengthens the skin and keeps it from becoming dry. Almond oil also increases the elasticity of the skin so it is less likely to tear.

Olive oil can also be used. Just mix some extra virgin olive oil with Aloe Vera gel and vitamins a and e in a blender or food processor and put the mixture in the fridge to cool before applying to the skin. Another option is to mix the olive oil with vitamin e oil, vanilla extract, cocoa butter and melted beeswax. This can also be cooled in the fridge before massaging or having someone else massage it into the skin.

After the baby is born it is safe to use Retin A creams and lotions to treat any stretch marks that developed but do not use them while pregnant or if you are nursing.

Stretch Marks and Teenagers

Teenagers have to endure many changes to their bodies because of puberty and the hormonal changes that accompany it. They suffer through acne, boys voices change, girls develop breasts and they all fight to understand feelings that they have never experienced before. At this point in their lives all teens want to fit in and not stand out for any reason.

Unfortunately, puberty is often accompanied by growth spurts and hormonal changes and this combination usually results in unsightly stretch marks. Boys get them on their backs and shoulders while the girls get them on their hips, thighs and breasts. Because of their age and the general elasticity of their skin teenagers have the best chance of healing stretch marks and so, if they are feeling self conscious about their marks they should start a treatment regimen as soon as possible after the marks appear. Teenagers can use the creams, oils and lotions recommended for dealing with stretch marks or ones designed to remove scars. It is important to apply these creams several times a day.

If teenagers want to avoid getting stretch marks they should first pay close attention to what they eat. A balanced diet that contains ample amounts of vitamins and minerals will help in keeping the skin supple and elastic. It will also ensure that enough collagen is being produced. Vitamins also assist in the repair of tissues Teens should avoid drastic diets that lead to rapid weight gain on loss in a short period of time. Getting lots of exercise also helps as it prevents weight gain.

Because of the age of teenagers treatments such as surgery are probably not recommended because their bodies are still changing.

Stretch Marks – They're not Just for

Women

When most people think of stretch marks they think first of pregnant women but while it is true that many expectant mothers find themselves dealing with the development of stretch marks, men are not immune to the unsightly scars. Just as with women some men are more prone to getting stretch marks than others. And just like women most men who get stretch marks would like to get rid of them or at least reduce the appearance of stretch marks.

Many men who get stretch marks often get them as a result of rapid muscle growth from weight training or other forms of exercise. Men naturally build muscle faster than women so for men who can't resist the temptation to "bulk up' as quickly as possible ending up with stretch marks is a real possibility. They are even more at risk if they are body builders and others who take supplements to enhance their workouts as the hormones present in these supplements have been shown to add to the risk of developing stretch marks and also increase the rate of muscle development. Many male athletes also use medications containing corticosteroids to treat injuries because it reduces inflammation and accelerates healing but corticosteroids have also been tied to the appearance of stretch marks. Teenage boys also tend to experience growth spurts that can lead to development of stretch marks.

In men stretch marks usually appear on the upper arms, under arms, shoulders, back and thighs as these are the areas that expand the most as a result on lifting weights. They are often less noticeable than women's but only because men generally have more hair on their bodies than women do. However for many athletes and especially body builders this is no comfort because they shave their bodies for competitions.

You might think that something harmless like stretch marks would not bother a man but the reality is that many men are very embarrassed or self-conscious about their stretch and want to get rid of them. The tip to avoiding stretch marks for these men is to use lighter weights and to build muscle more gradually using more reps instead so the skin does not have to stretch as far as fast. Keeping skin moisturized and the body hydrated also helps in avoiding stretch marks and in treating them when they appear. Some of the creams used to treat stretch marks can be found in the skin ailment aisle rather than having to go to the makeup and skin care counter so men might feel more comfortable buying these. There are also stretch mark creams that are unscented so men can make use of those options without feeling self-conscious.

summarize

To summarize what we have discussed, Stretch marks are formed when the skin is stretch too far too quickly and it tears leaving red angry scars called stretch marks. Recent studies have found that the presence of certain hormones can also contribute to the development of stretch marks. Everyone can get stretch marks and once you get them they are there to stay. Despite their permanence stretch marks do not pose a health risk and they are not painful, although they might itch a little. They also do not stay red or purple but fade over time to a silvery or white color.

Although everyone is susceptible to stretch marks they are most often found on pregnant women, body builders or people who train with heavy weights and use supplements, and people who have either gained or lost and regained significant weight in a relatively short period of time.

Although they do not completely disappear the appearance of stretch marks can be reduced and there are many creams, oils and lotions on the market that claim. They have varying degrees of success and there are also homemade versions that can have the same effect for much less money. For those who can afford it there is also the option of laser therapy and/or surgery to remove stretch marks.

So stretch marks are with us to stay at least until something new is invented to remove them. All you can do is to keep your skin as moisturized and supple as possible so that it retains its elasticity, try to maintain a steady weight, avoid rapid weight gain even when you are pregnant and hope for the best.

www.ingramcontent.com/pod-product-compliance
Lightning Source LLC
Chambersburg PA
CBHW080801310526
45791CB00030B/2937